SUNDAY	MONDAY	TUESDAY	WEDNESDAY	THURSDAY	FRIDAY	SATURDAY

NOTES

NOTES

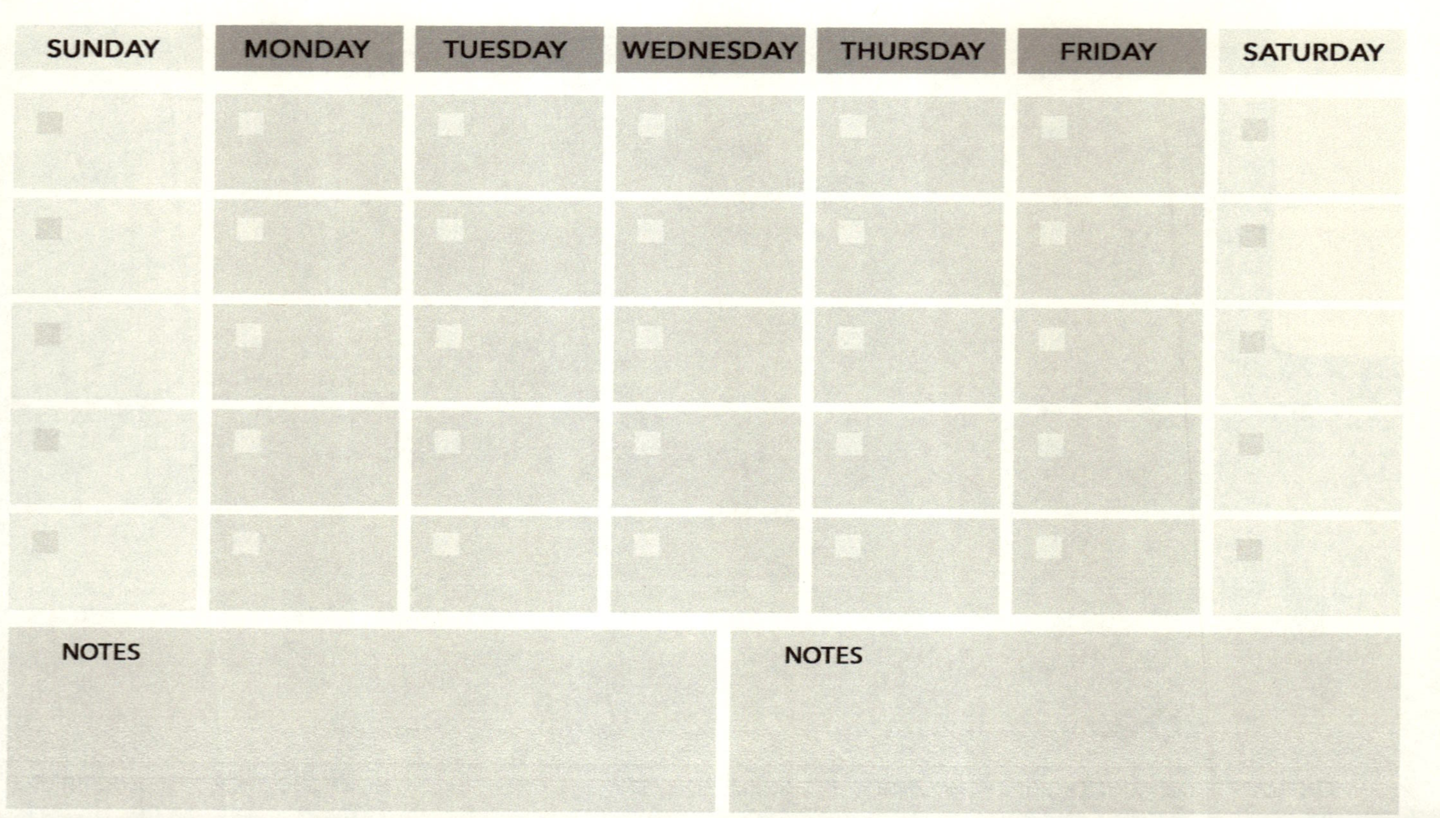

SUNDAY
MONDAY
TUESDAY
WEDNESDAY
THURSDAY
FRIDAY
SATURDAY
NOTES
NOTES

SUNDAY	MONDAY	TUESDAY	WEDNESDAY	THURSDAY	FRIDAY	SATURDAY

NOTES

NOTES

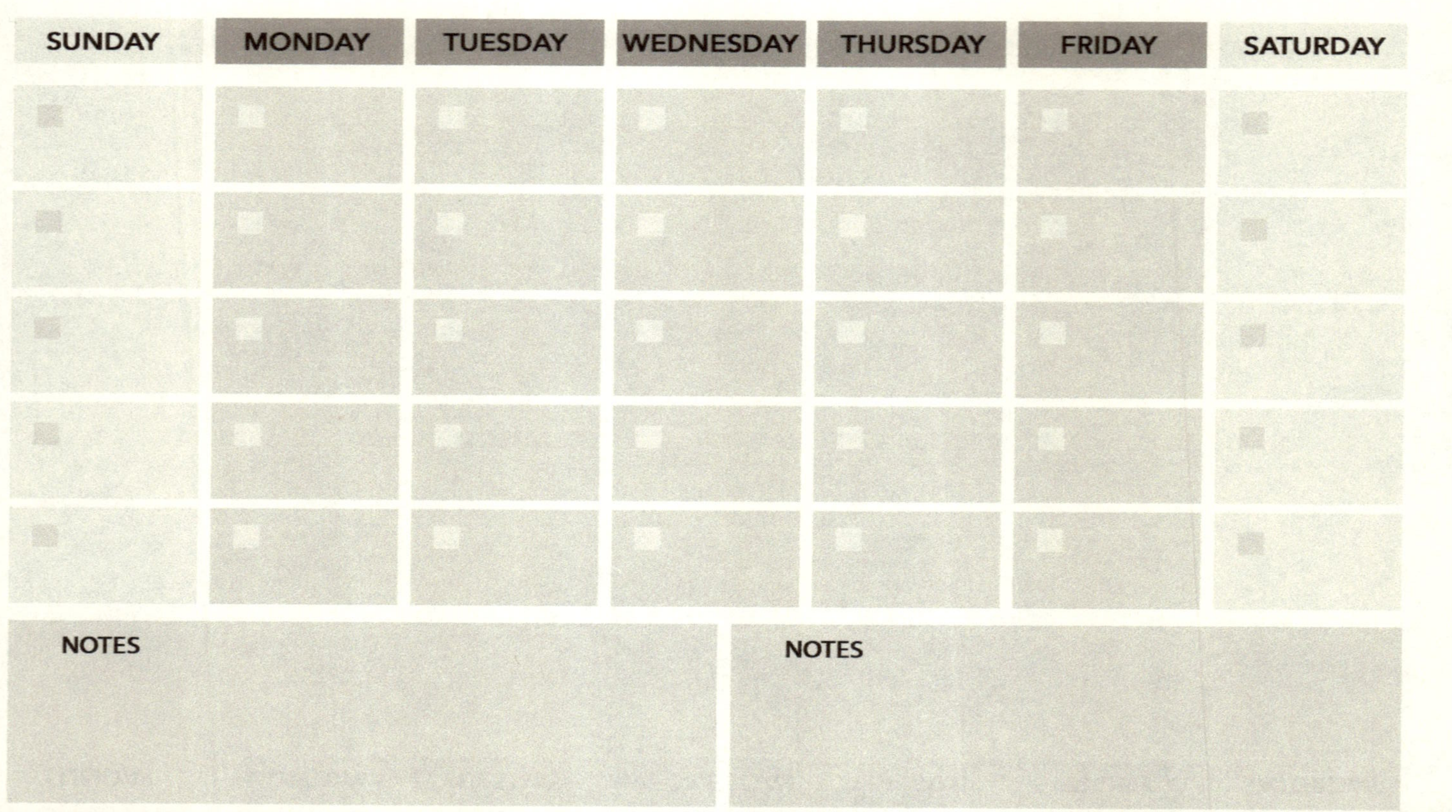

SUNDAY
MONDAY
TUESDAY
WEDNESDAY
THURSDAY
FRIDAY
SATURDAY
NOTES
NOTES

SUNDAY	MONDAY	TUESDAY	WEDNESDAY	THURSDAY	FRIDAY	SATURDAY

NOTES

NOTES

SUNDAY	MONDAY	TUESDAY	WEDNESDAY	THURSDAY	FRIDAY	SATURDAY

NOTES

NOTES

SUNDAY	MONDAY	TUESDAY	WEDNESDAY	THURSDAY	FRIDAY	SATURDAY

NOTES

NOTES

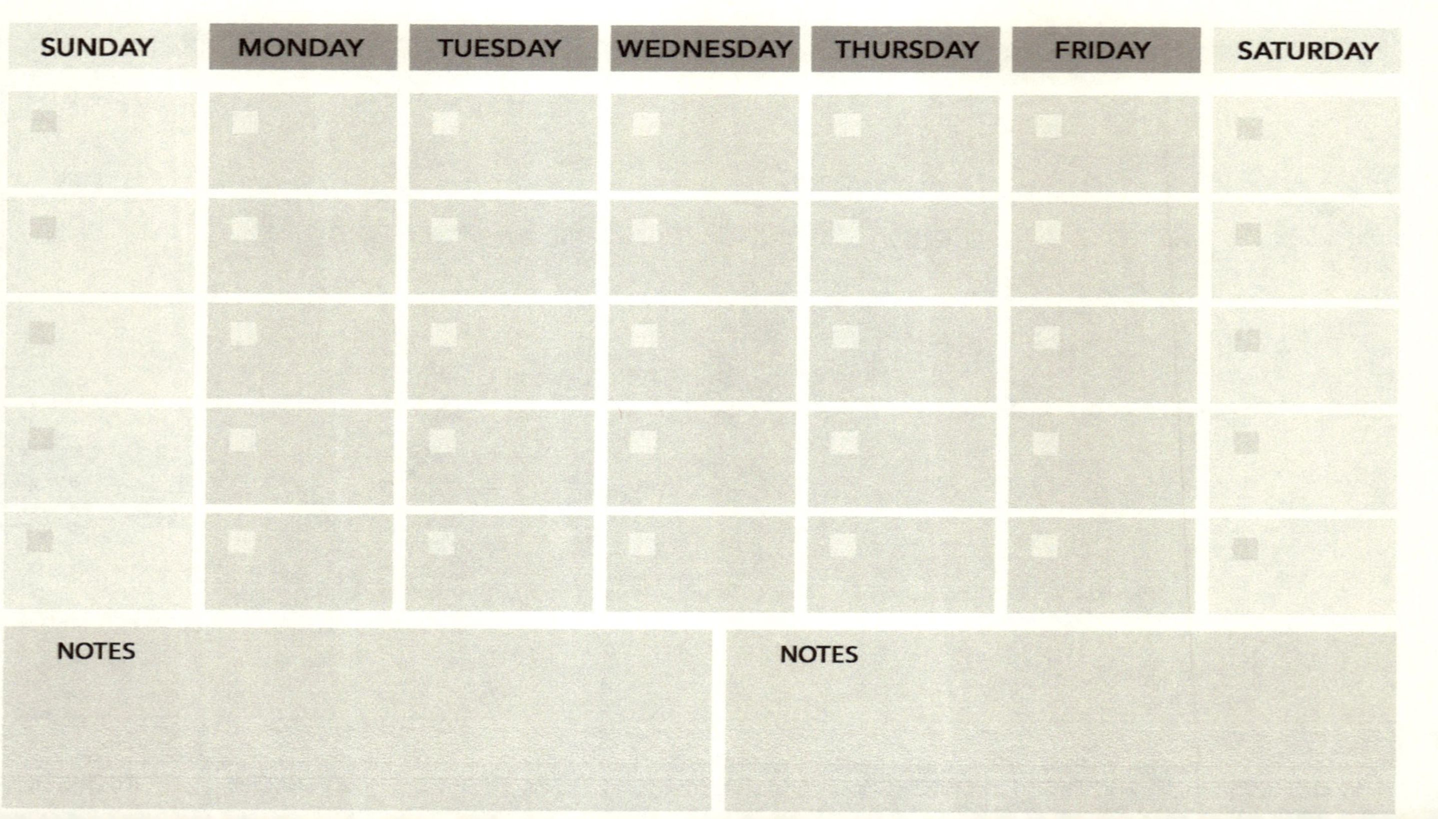

SUNDAY
MONDAY
TUESDAY
WEDNESDAY
THURSDAY
FRIDAY
SATURDAY
NOTES
NOTES

SUNDAY	MONDAY	TUESDAY	WEDNESDAY	THURSDAY	FRIDAY	SATURDAY

NOTES

NOTES

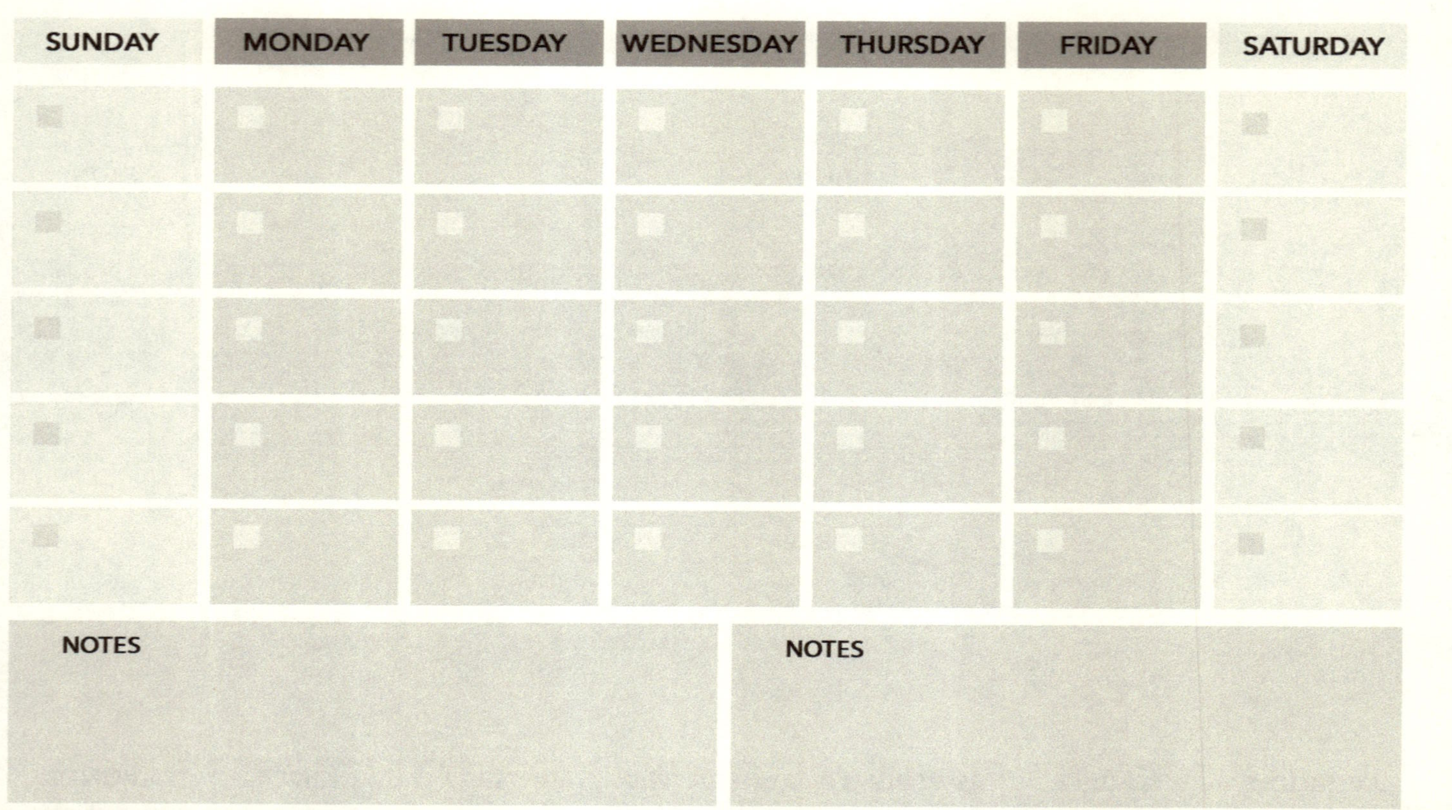

SUNDAY
MONDAY
TUESDAY
WEDNESDAY
THURSDAY
FRIDAY
SATURDAY
NOTES
NOTES

SUNDAY	MONDAY	TUESDAY	WEDNESDAY	THURSDAY	FRIDAY	SATURDAY

NOTES

NOTES

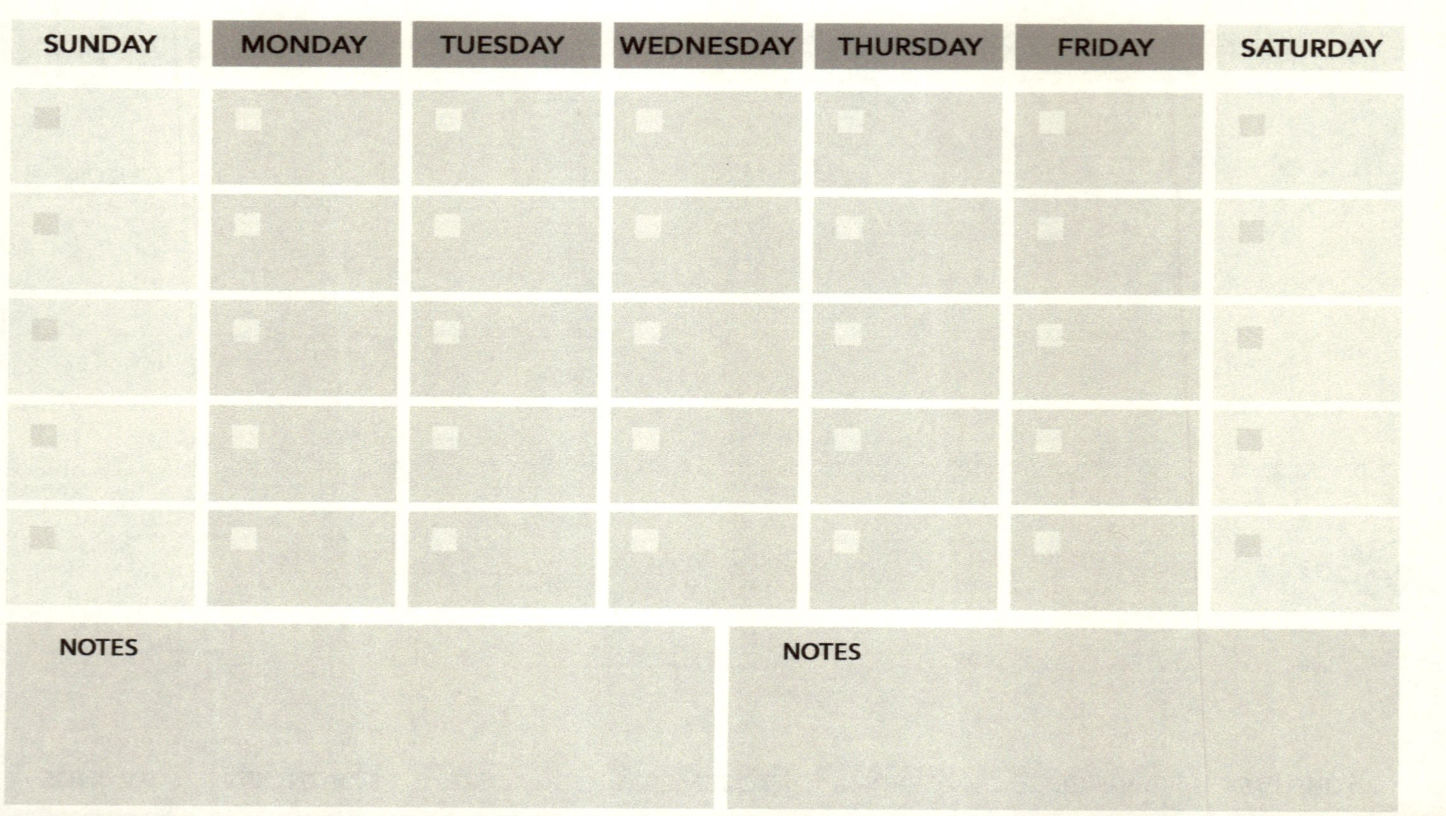

SUNDAY
MONDAY
TUESDAY
WEDNESDAY
THURSDAY
FRIDAY
SATURDAY
NOTES
NOTES

SUNDAY	MONDAY	TUESDAY	WEDNESDAY	THURSDAY	FRIDAY	SATURDAY

NOTES

NOTES

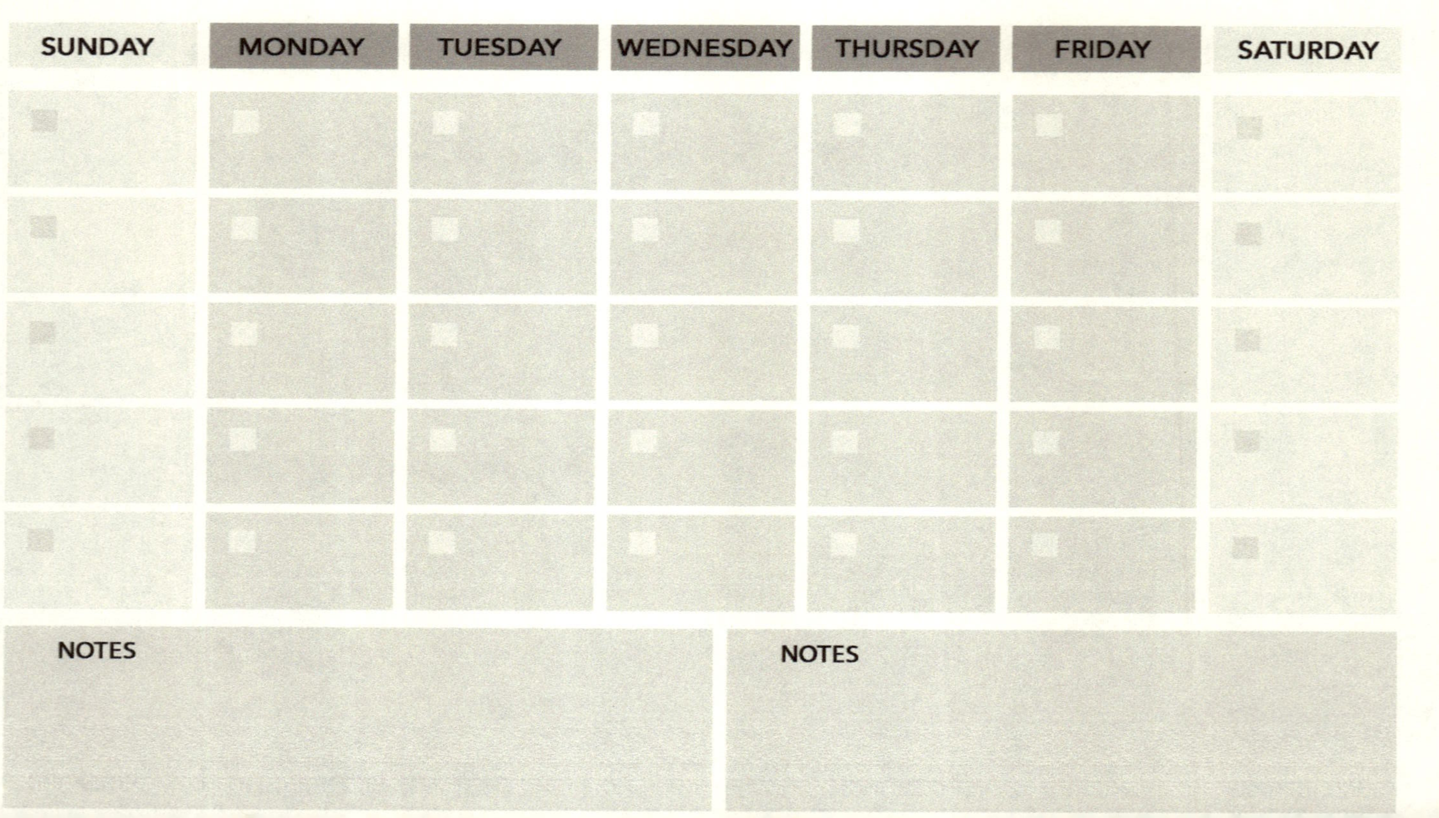

SUNDAY
MONDAY
TUESDAY
WEDNESDAY
THURSDAY
FRIDAY
SATURDAY
NOTES
NOTES

SUNDAY	MONDAY	TUESDAY	WEDNESDAY	THURSDAY	FRIDAY	SATURDAY

NOTES

NOTES

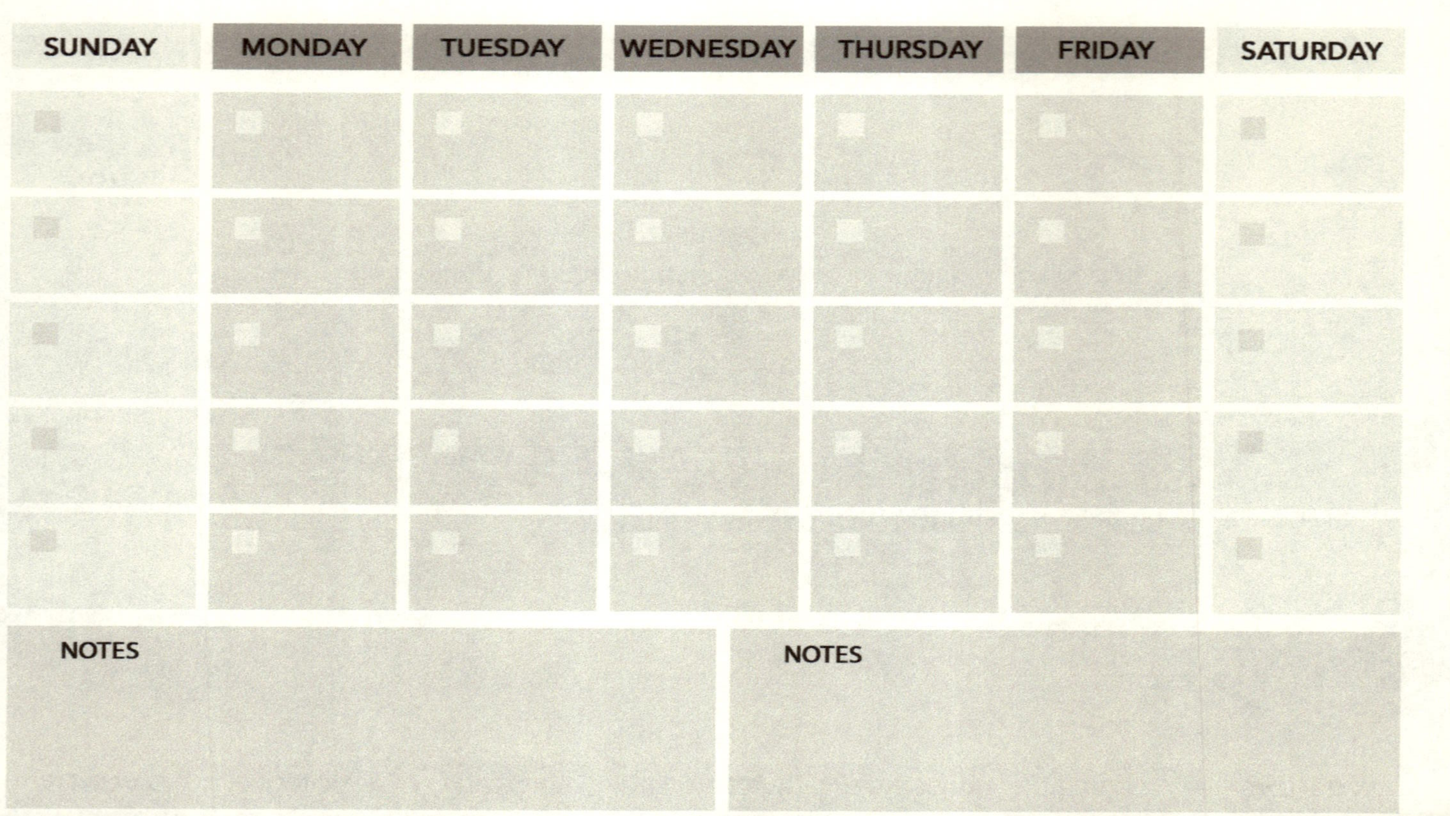

SUNDAY
MONDAY
TUESDAY
WEDNESDAY
THURSDAY
FRIDAY
SATURDAY
NOTES
NOTES

SUNDAY	MONDAY	TUESDAY	WEDNESDAY	THURSDAY	FRIDAY	SATURDAY

NOTES

NOTES

SUNDAY	MONDAY	TUESDAY	WEDNESDAY	THURSDAY	FRIDAY	SATURDAY

NOTES

NOTES

SUNDAY	MONDAY	TUESDAY	WEDNESDAY	THURSDAY	FRIDAY	SATURDAY

NOTES

NOTES

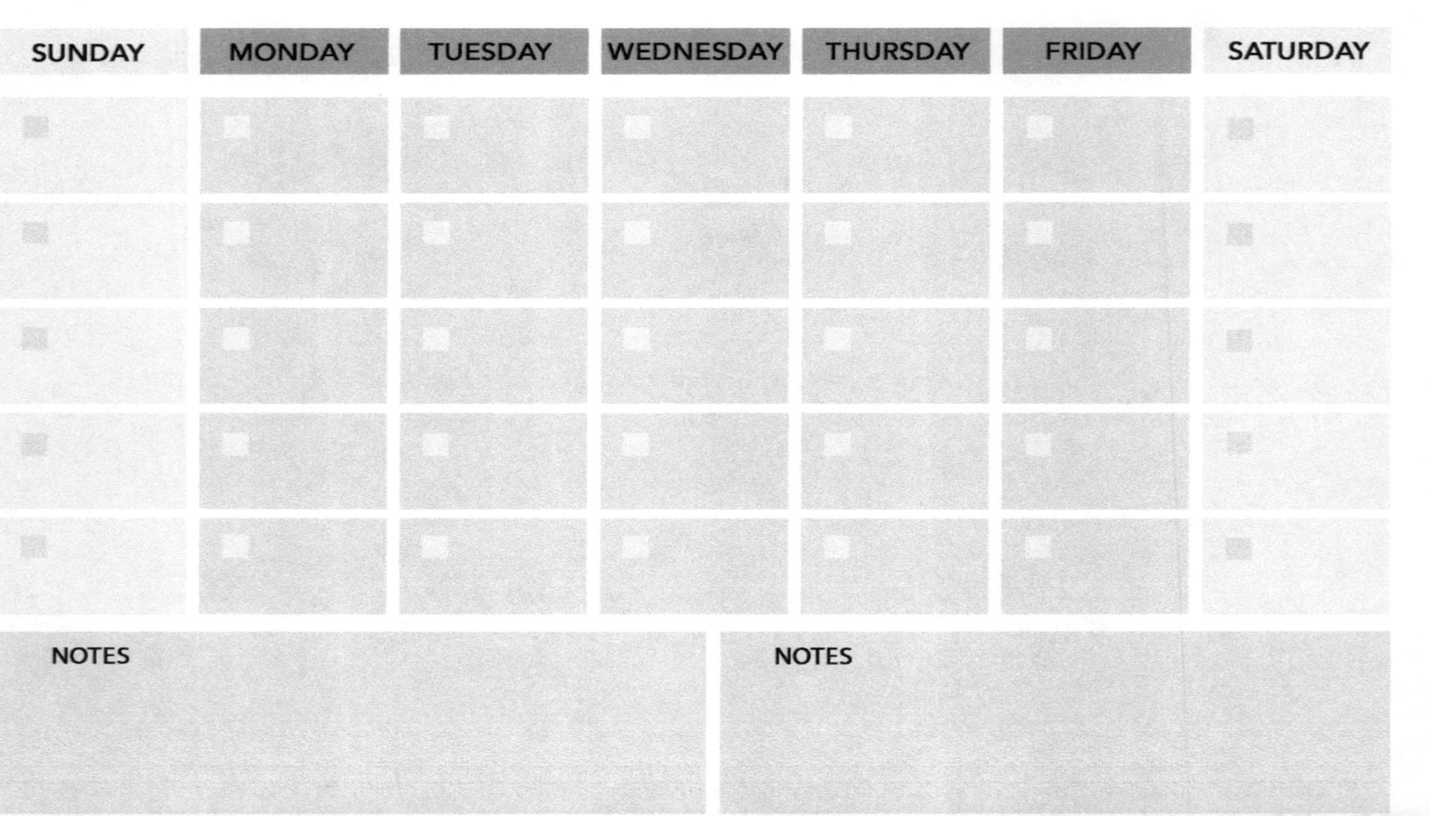

SUNDAY
MONDAY
TUESDAY
WEDNESDAY
THURSDAY
FRIDAY
SATURDAY
NOTES
NOTES

SUNDAY	MONDAY	TUESDAY	WEDNESDAY	THURSDAY	FRIDAY	SATURDAY

NOTES

NOTES

SUNDAY	MONDAY	TUESDAY	WEDNESDAY	THURSDAY	FRIDAY	SATURDAY

NOTES

NOTES

SUNDAY	MONDAY	TUESDAY	WEDNESDAY	THURSDAY	FRIDAY	SATURDAY

NOTES

NOTES

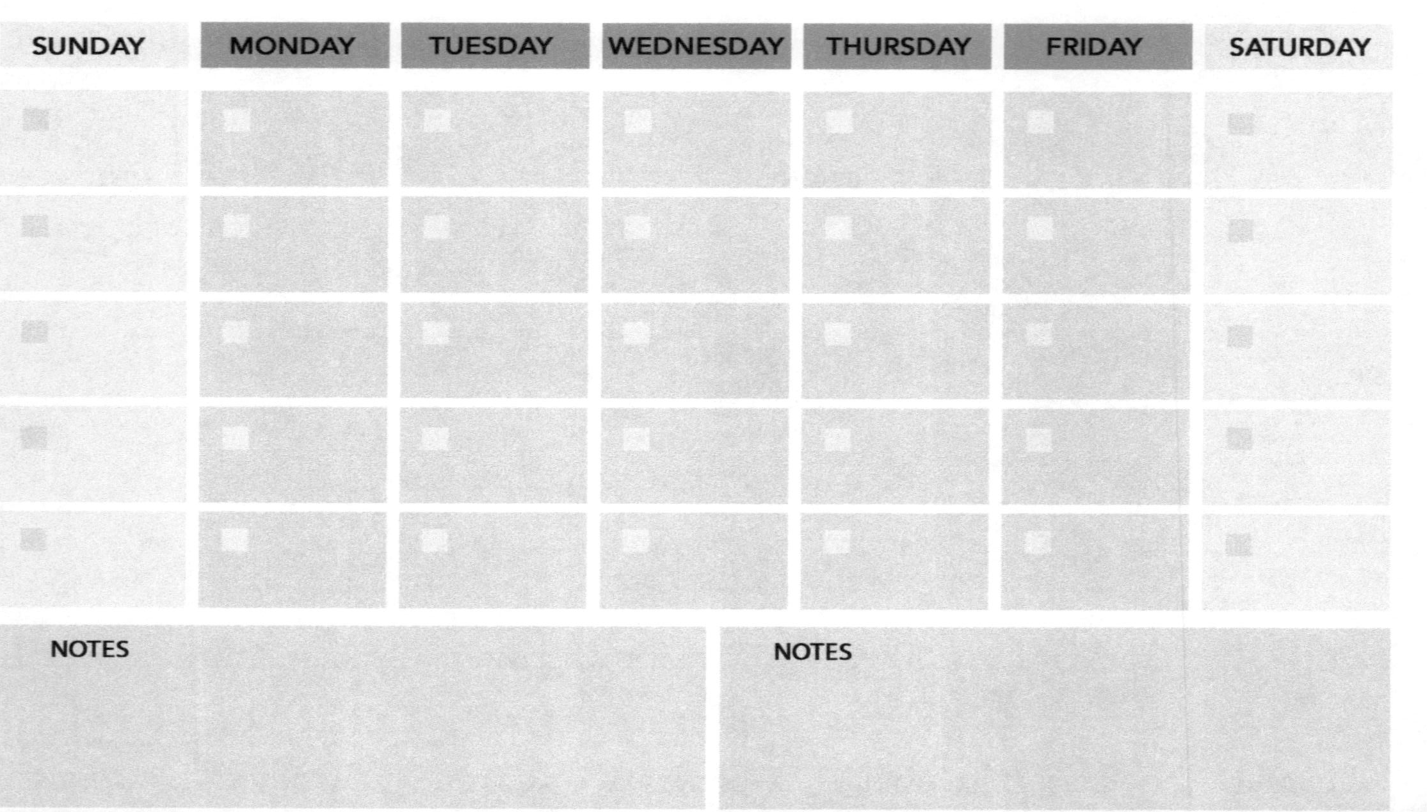

SUNDAY
MONDAY
TUESDAY
WEDNESDAY
THURSDAY
FRIDAY
SATURDAY
NOTES
NOTES

SUNDAY	MONDAY	TUESDAY	WEDNESDAY	THURSDAY	FRIDAY	SATURDAY

NOTES

NOTES

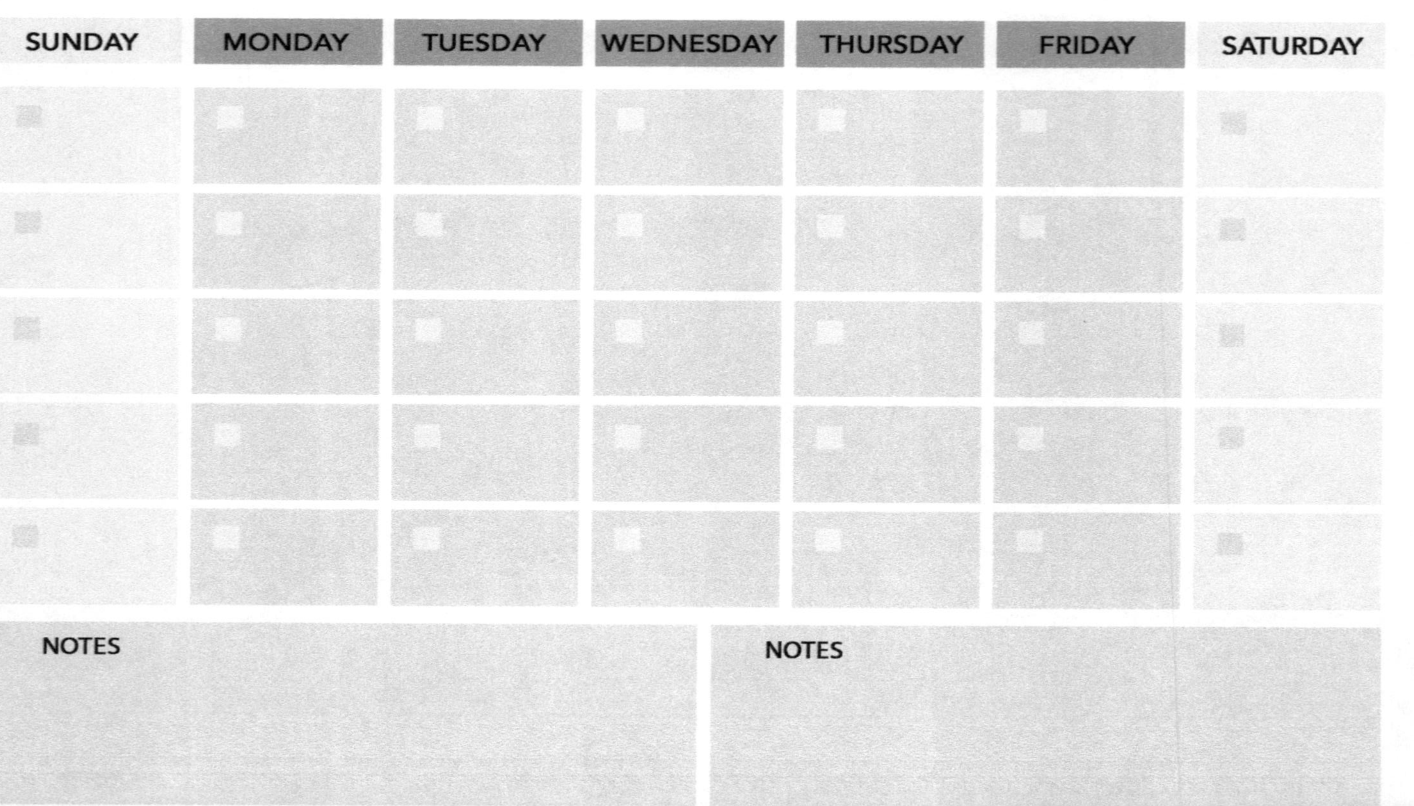

SUNDAY
MONDAY
TUESDAY
WEDNESDAY
THURSDAY
FRIDAY
SATURDAY
NOTES
NOTES

SUNDAY	MONDAY	TUESDAY	WEDNESDAY	THURSDAY	FRIDAY	SATURDAY

NOTES

NOTES

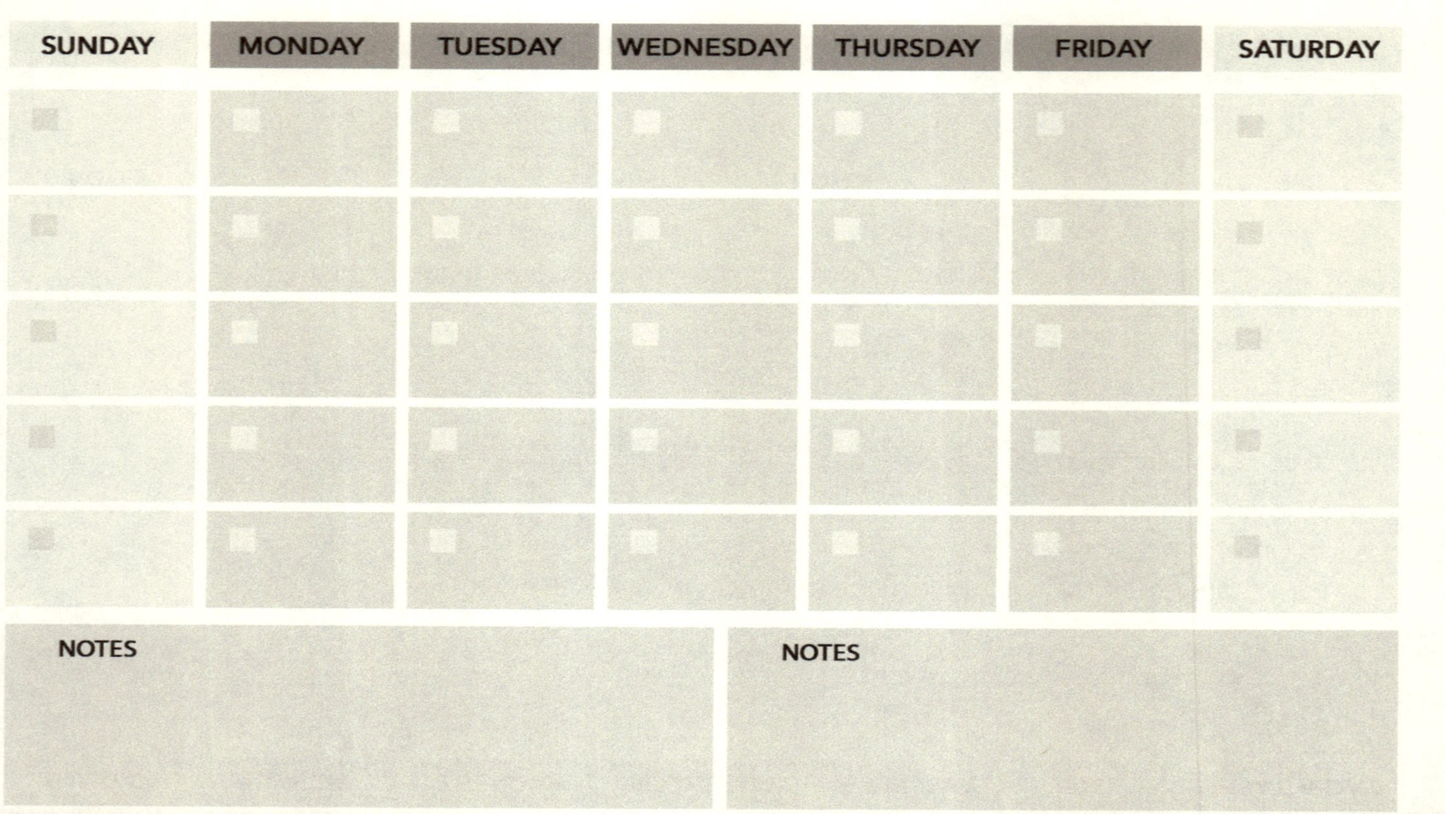
SUNDAY
MONDAY
TUESDAY
WEDNESDAY
THURSDAY
FRIDAY
SATURDAY
NOTES
NOTES

SUNDAY	MONDAY	TUESDAY	WEDNESDAY	THURSDAY	FRIDAY	SATURDAY

NOTES

NOTES

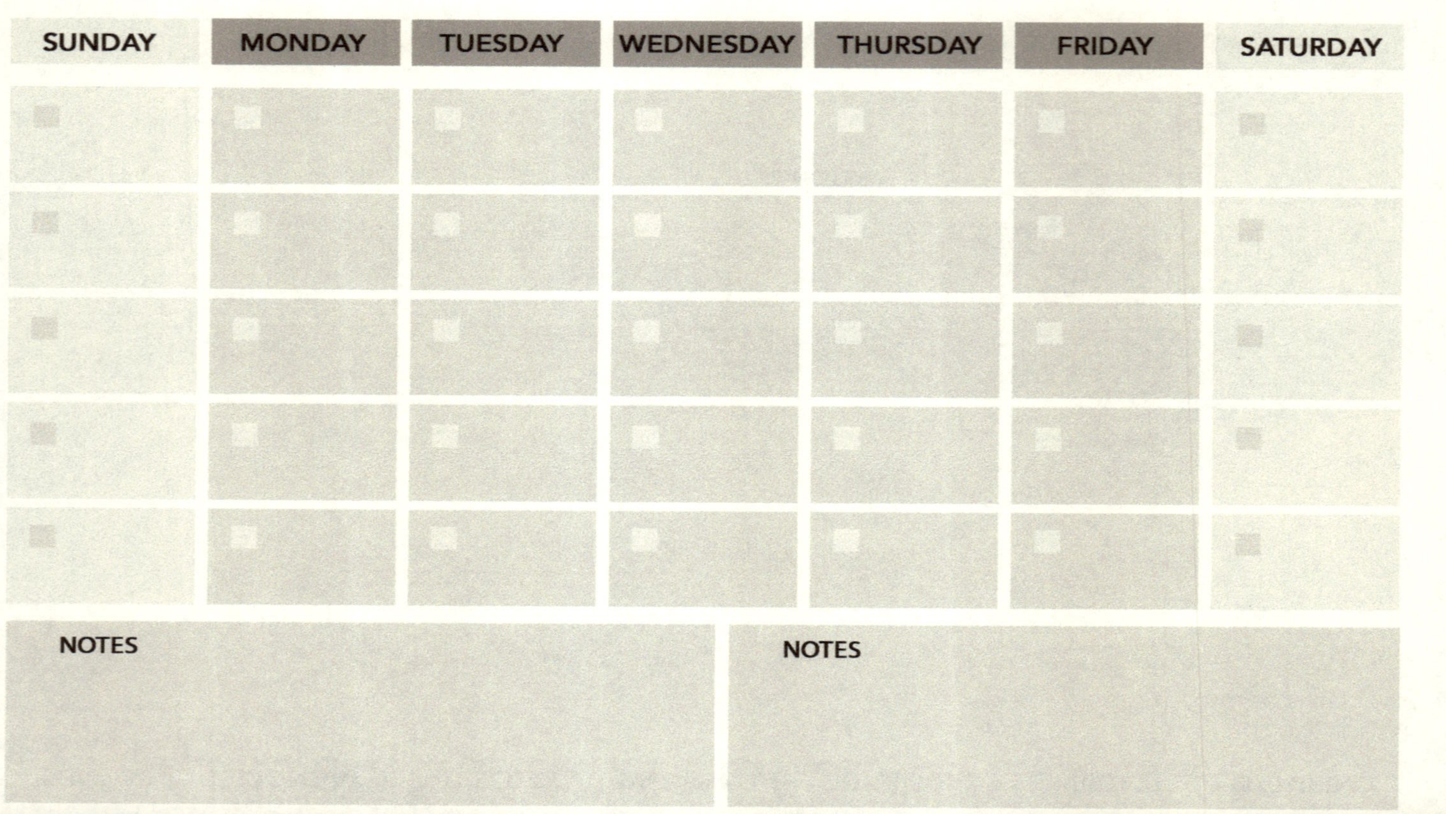

SUNDAY
MONDAY
TUESDAY
WEDNESDAY
THURSDAY
FRIDAY
SATURDAY
NOTES
NOTES

SUNDAY	MONDAY	TUESDAY	WEDNESDAY	THURSDAY	FRIDAY	SATURDAY

NOTES

NOTES

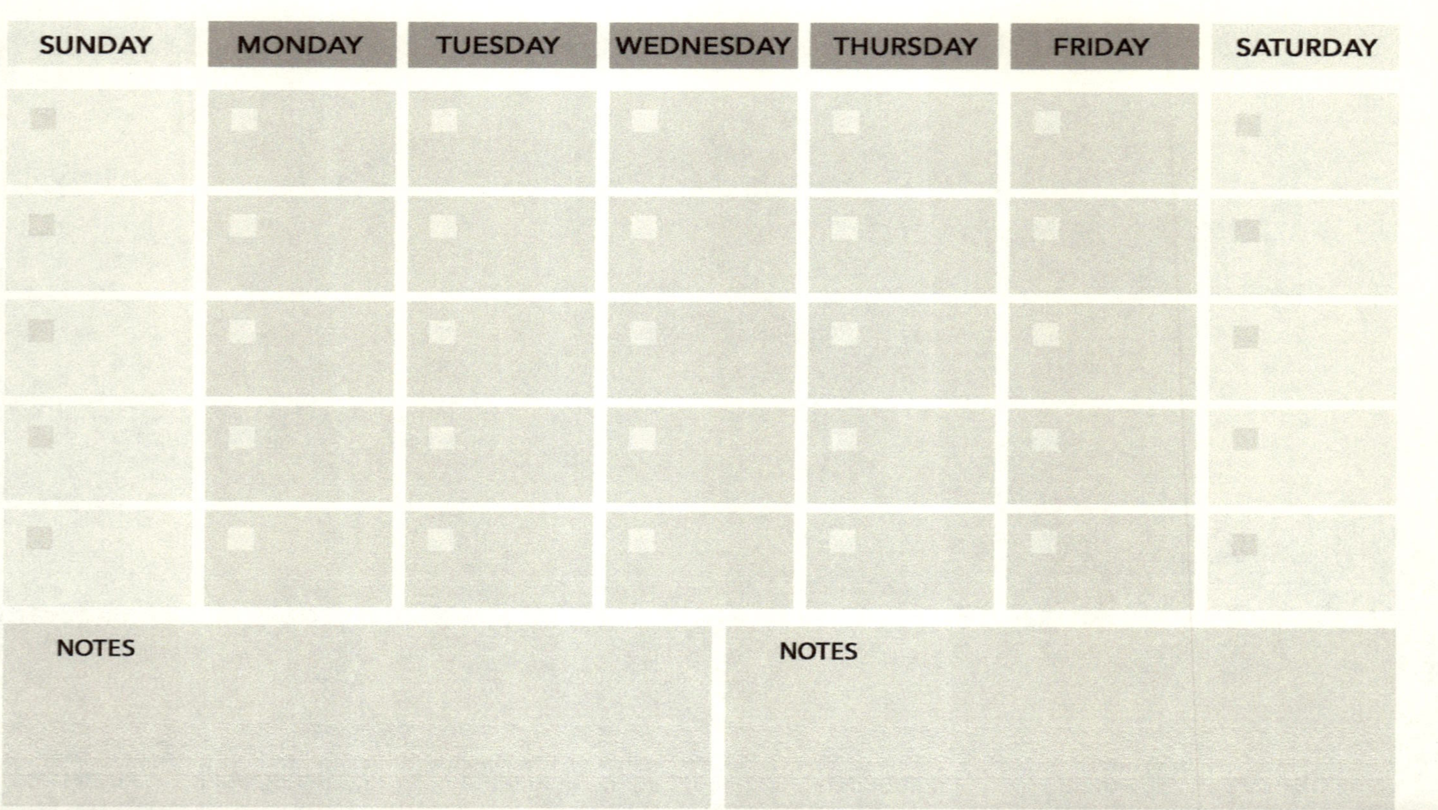

SUNDAY
MONDAY
TUESDAY
WEDNESDAY
THURSDAY
FRIDAY
SATURDAY
NOTES
NOTES

SUNDAY	MONDAY	TUESDAY	WEDNESDAY	THURSDAY	FRIDAY	SATURDAY

NOTES

NOTES

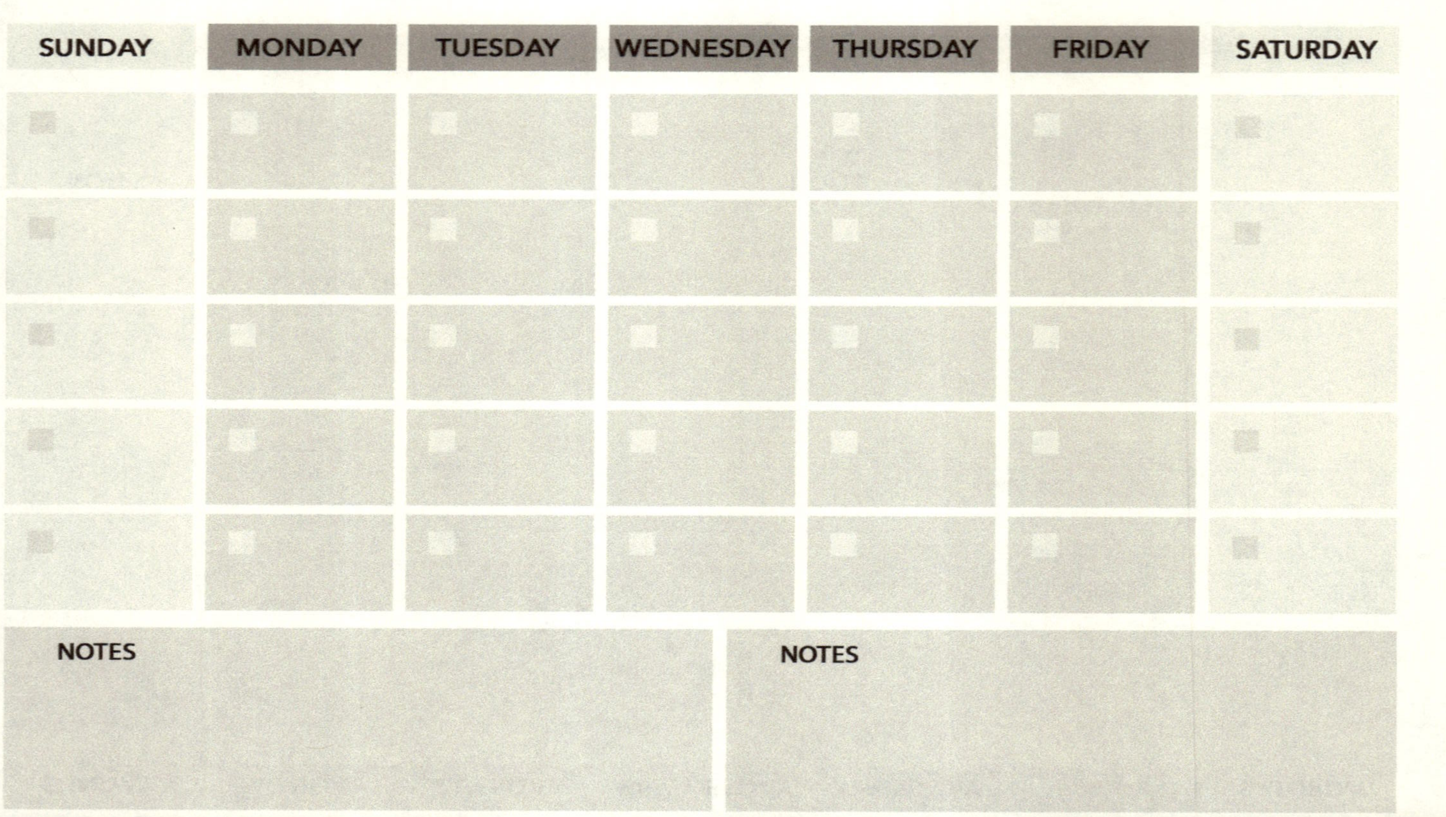

SUNDAY
MONDAY
TUESDAY
WEDNESDAY
THURSDAY
FRIDAY
SATURDAY
NOTES
NOTES

SUNDAY	MONDAY	TUESDAY	WEDNESDAY	THURSDAY	FRIDAY	SATURDAY

NOTES

NOTES

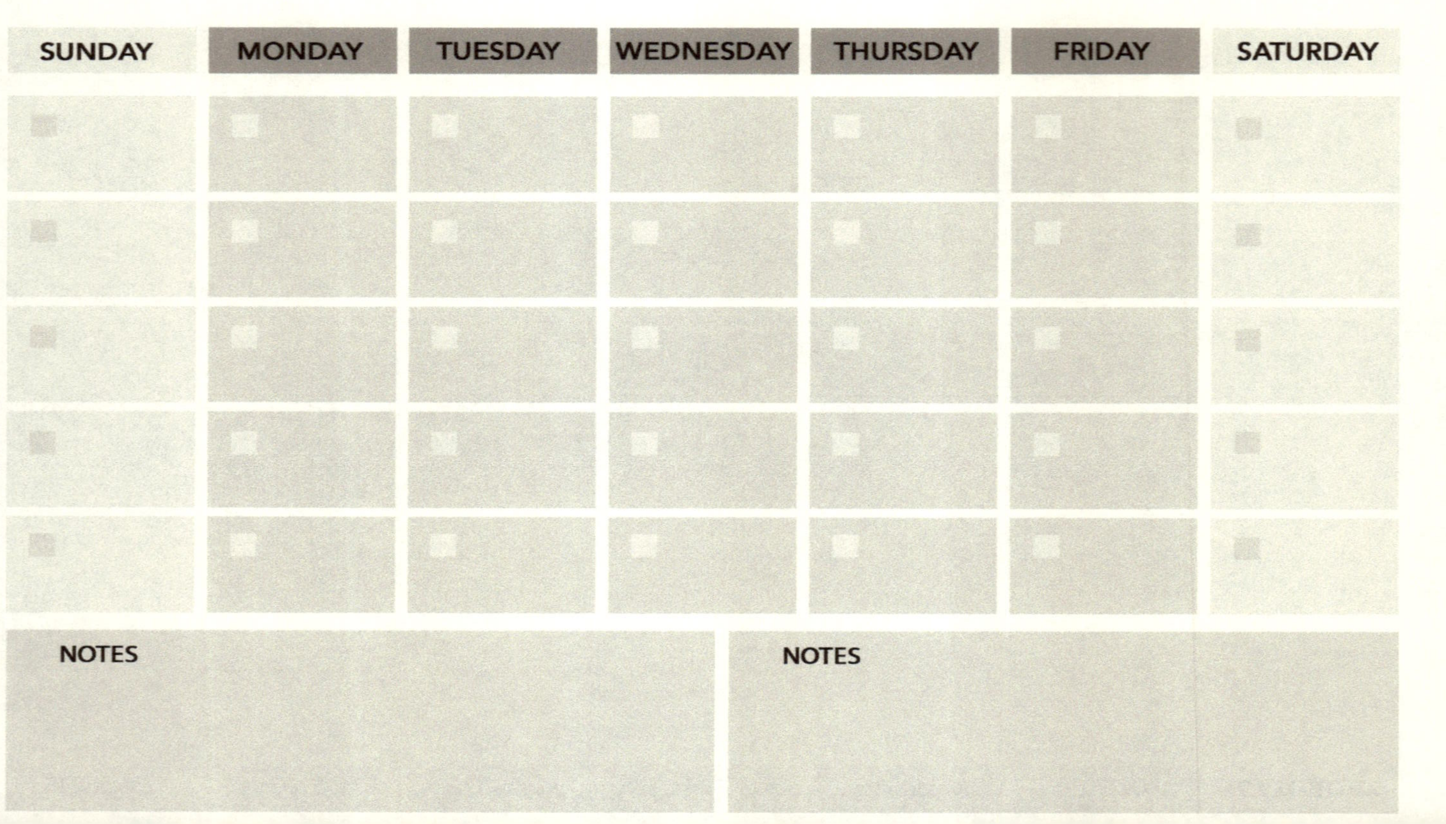

SUNDAY
MONDAY
TUESDAY
WEDNESDAY
THURSDAY
FRIDAY
SATURDAY
NOTES
NOTES

SUNDAY	MONDAY	TUESDAY	WEDNESDAY	THURSDAY	FRIDAY	SATURDAY

NOTES

NOTES

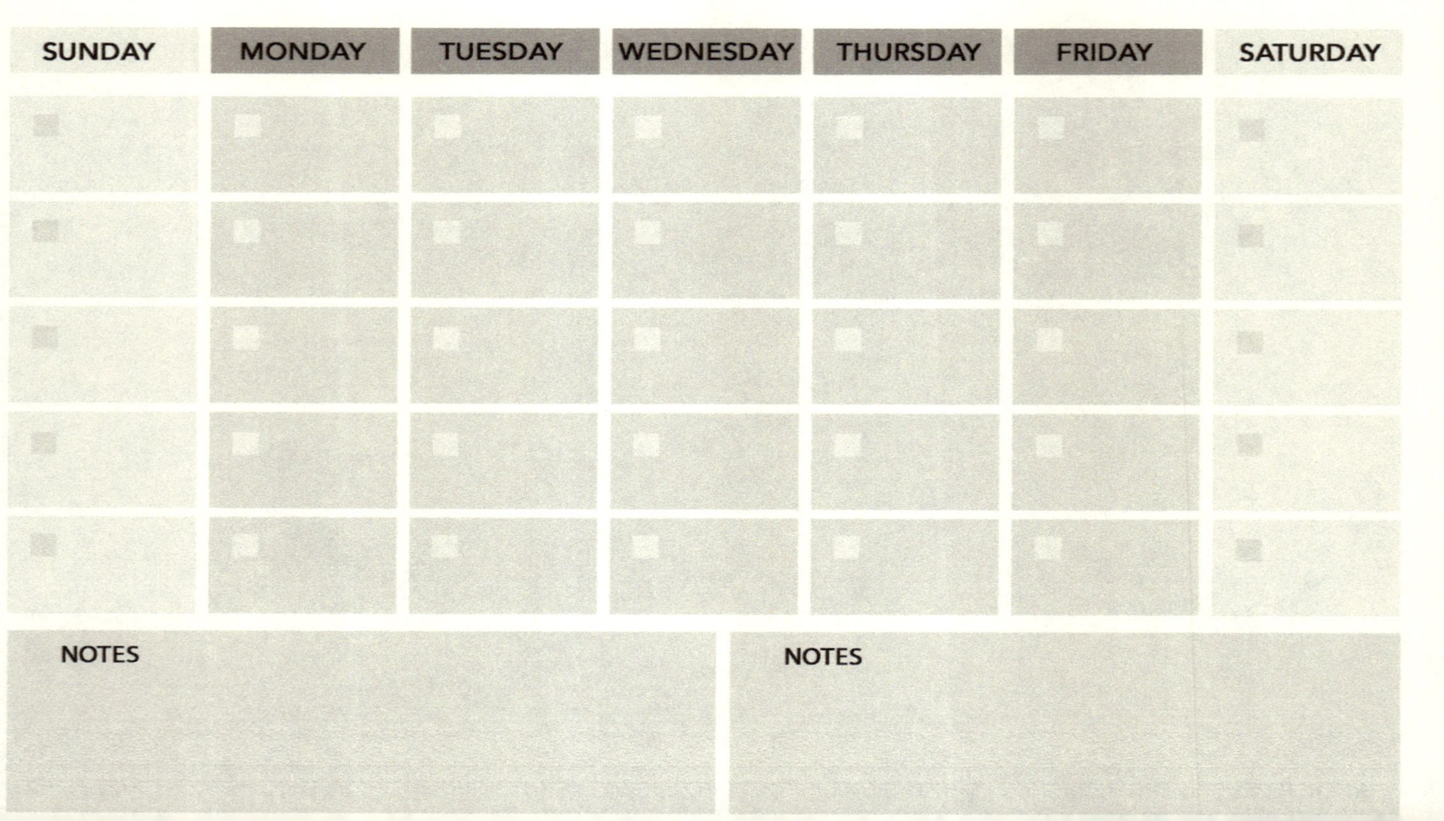

SUNDAY
MONDAY
TUESDAY
WEDNESDAY
THURSDAY
FRIDAY
SATURDAY
NOTES
NOTES

SUNDAY	MONDAY	TUESDAY	WEDNESDAY	THURSDAY	FRIDAY	SATURDAY

NOTES

NOTES

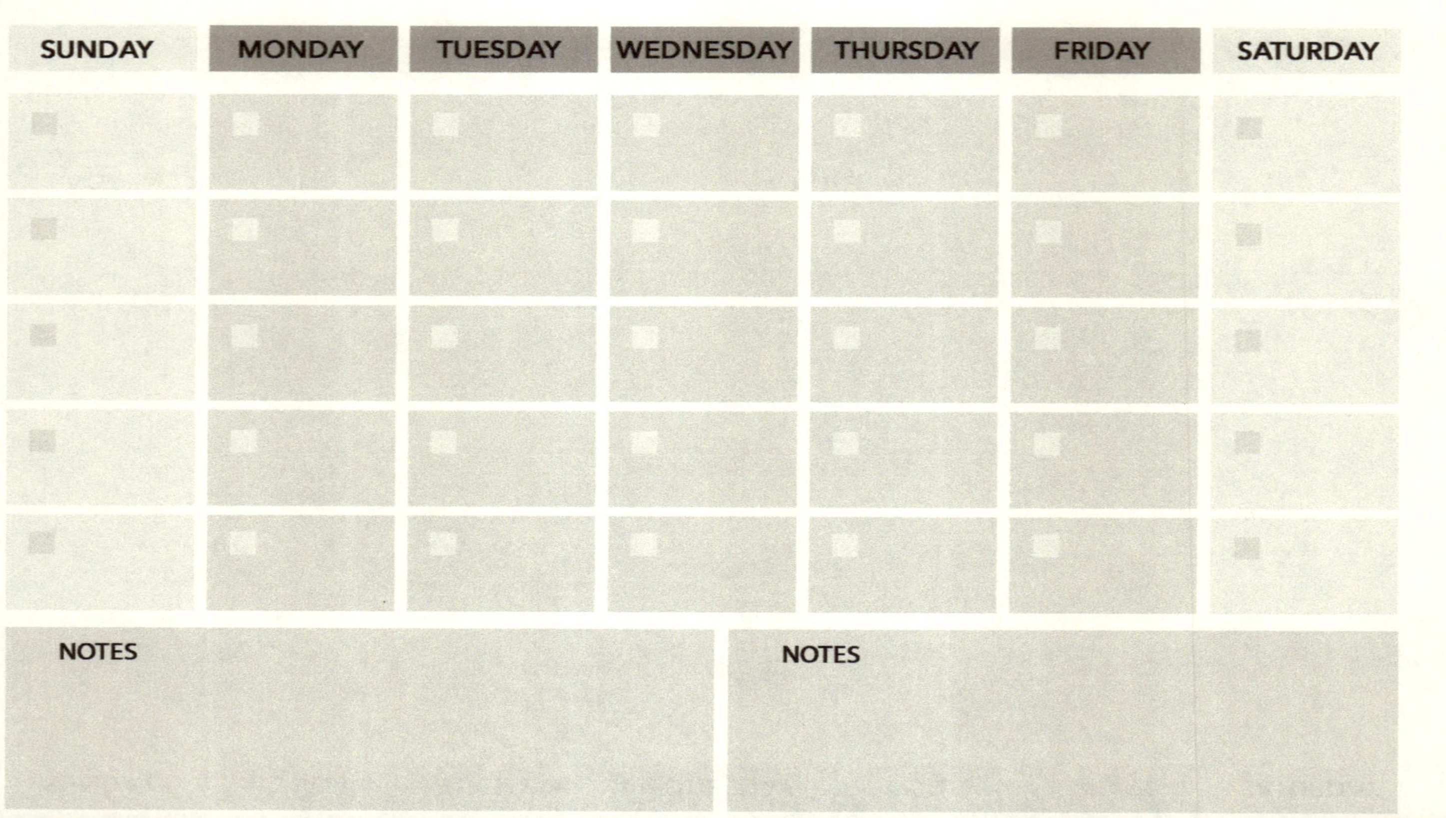

SUNDAY
MONDAY
TUESDAY
WEDNESDAY
THURSDAY
FRIDAY
SATURDAY
NOTES
NOTES

SUNDAY	MONDAY	TUESDAY	WEDNESDAY	THURSDAY	FRIDAY	SATURDAY

NOTES

NOTES

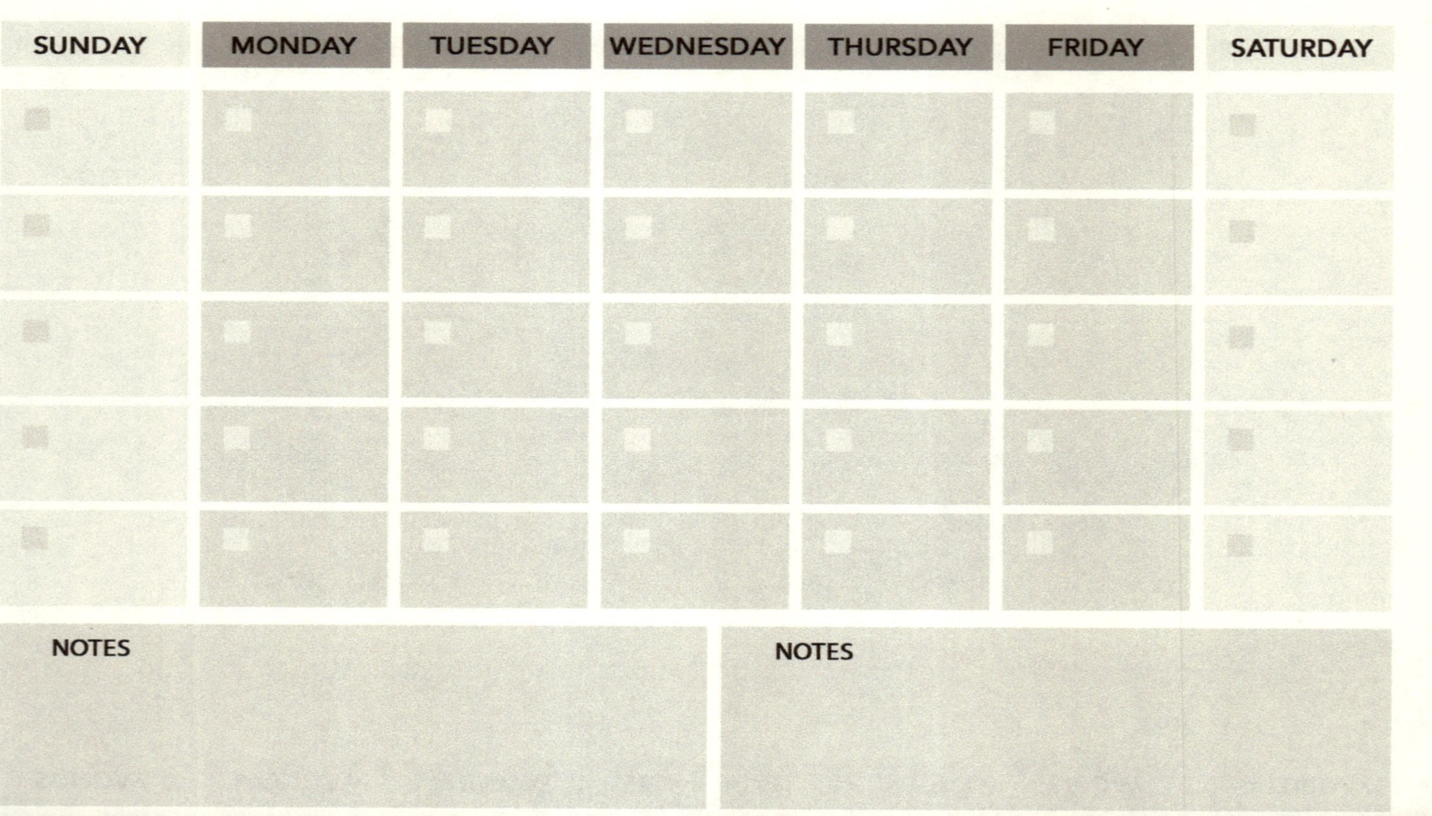

SUNDAY
MONDAY
TUESDAY
WEDNESDAY
THURSDAY
FRIDAY
SATURDAY
NOTES
NOTES

SUNDAY	MONDAY	TUESDAY	WEDNESDAY	THURSDAY	FRIDAY	SATURDAY

NOTES

NOTES

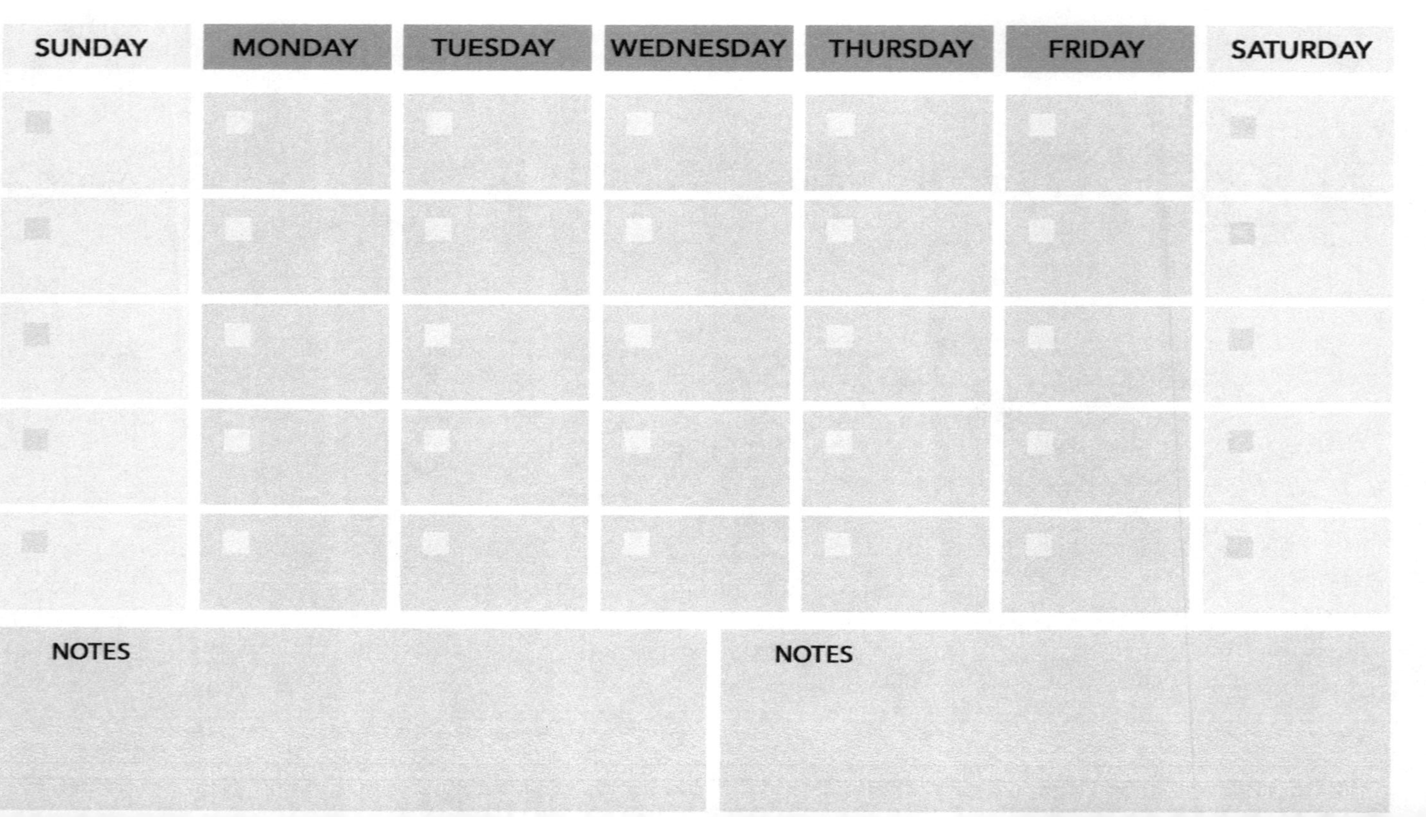

SUNDAY	MONDAY	TUESDAY	WEDNESDAY	THURSDAY	FRIDAY	SATURDAY

NOTES

NOTES

SUNDAY	MONDAY	TUESDAY	WEDNESDAY	THURSDAY	FRIDAY	SATURDAY

NOTES

NOTES

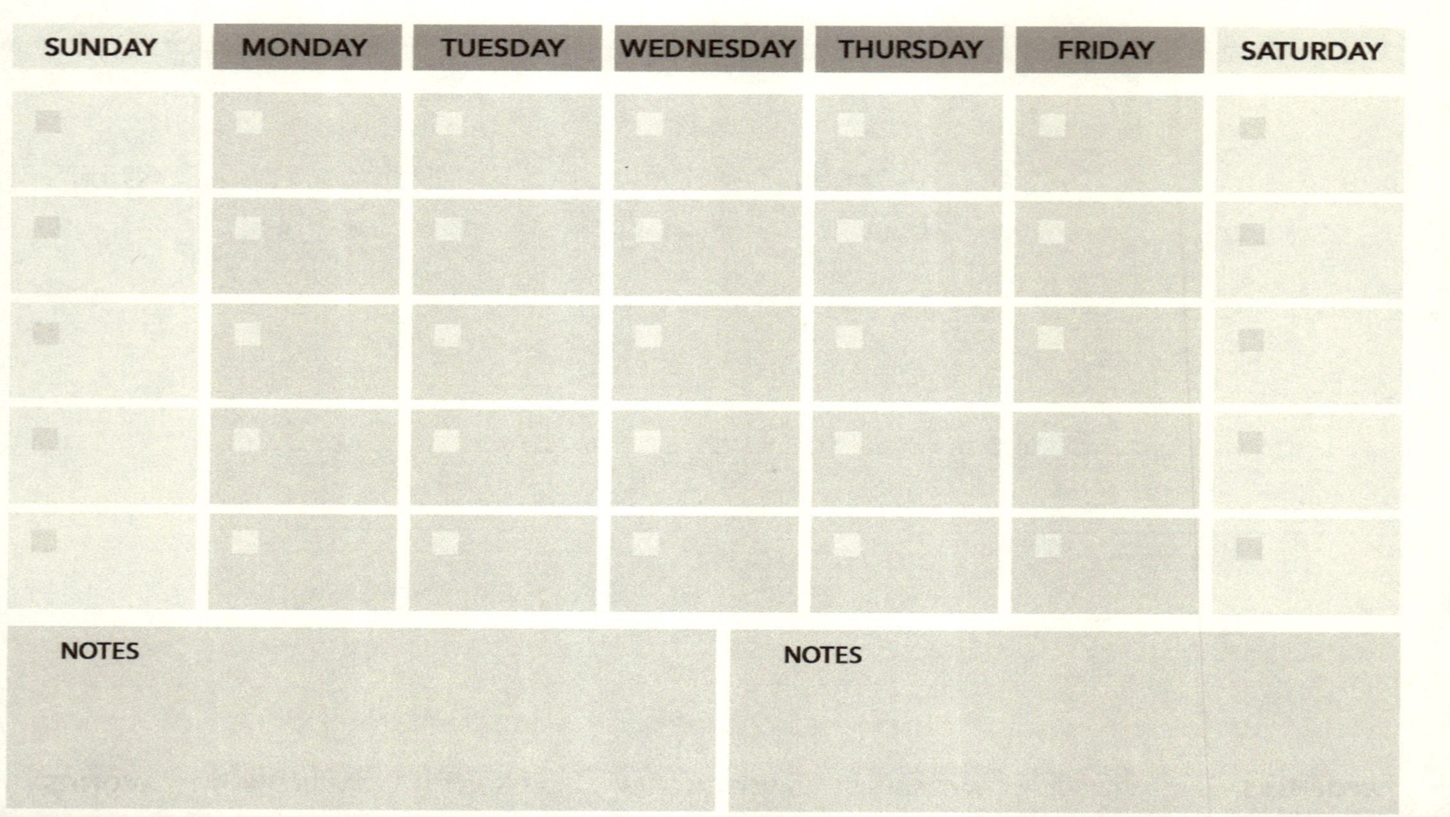

SUNDAY
MONDAY
TUESDAY
WEDNESDAY
THURSDAY
FRIDAY
SATURDAY
NOTES
NOTES

SUNDAY	MONDAY	TUESDAY	WEDNESDAY	THURSDAY	FRIDAY	SATURDAY

NOTES

NOTES

SUNDAY	MONDAY	TUESDAY	WEDNESDAY	THURSDAY	FRIDAY	SATURDAY

NOTES

NOTES

SUNDAY	MONDAY	TUESDAY	WEDNESDAY	THURSDAY	FRIDAY	SATURDAY

NOTES

NOTES

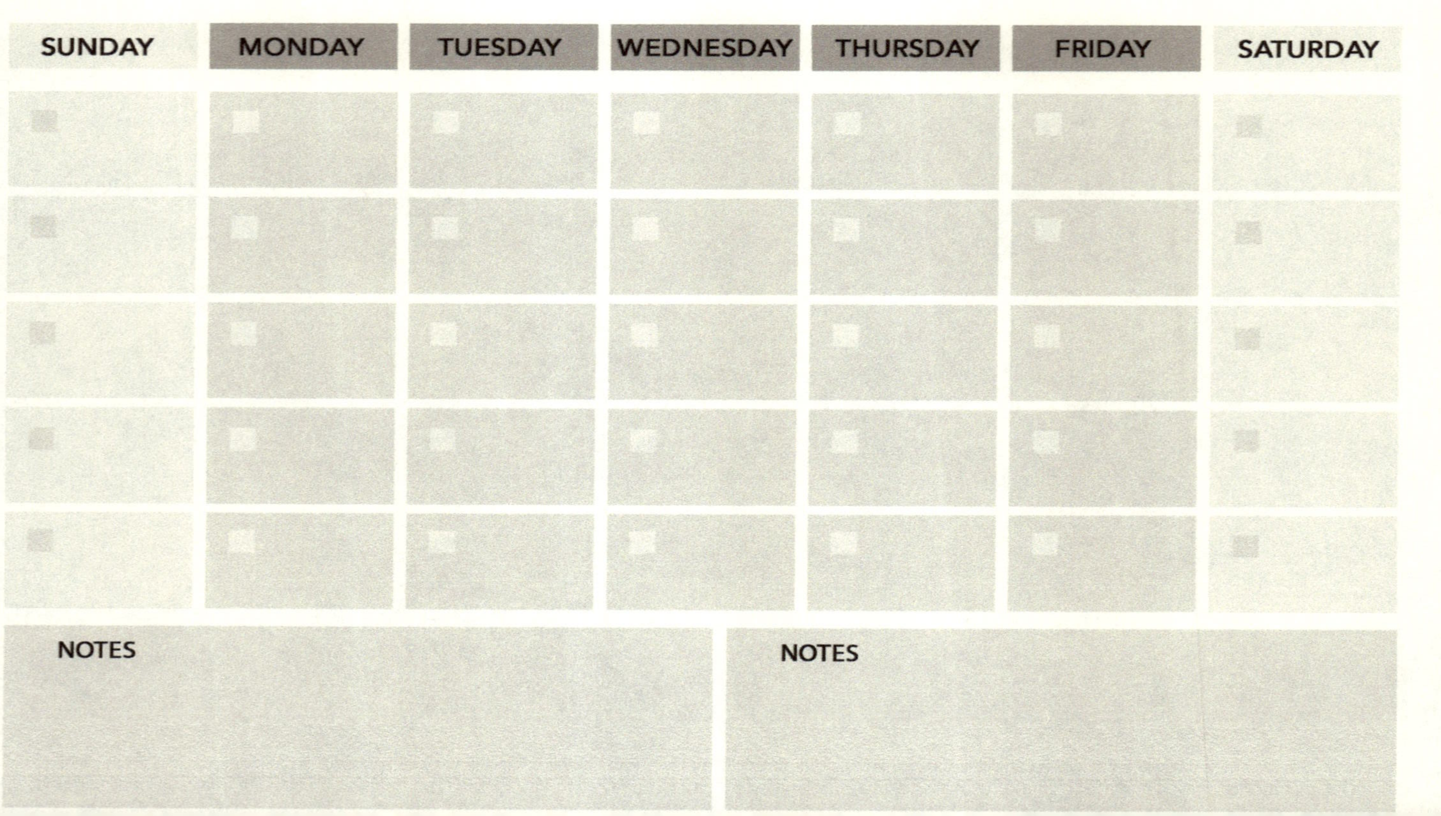

SUNDAY
MONDAY
TUESDAY
WEDNESDAY
THURSDAY
FRIDAY
SATURDAY
NOTES
NOTES

SUNDAY	MONDAY	TUESDAY	WEDNESDAY	THURSDAY	FRIDAY	SATURDAY

NOTES

NOTES

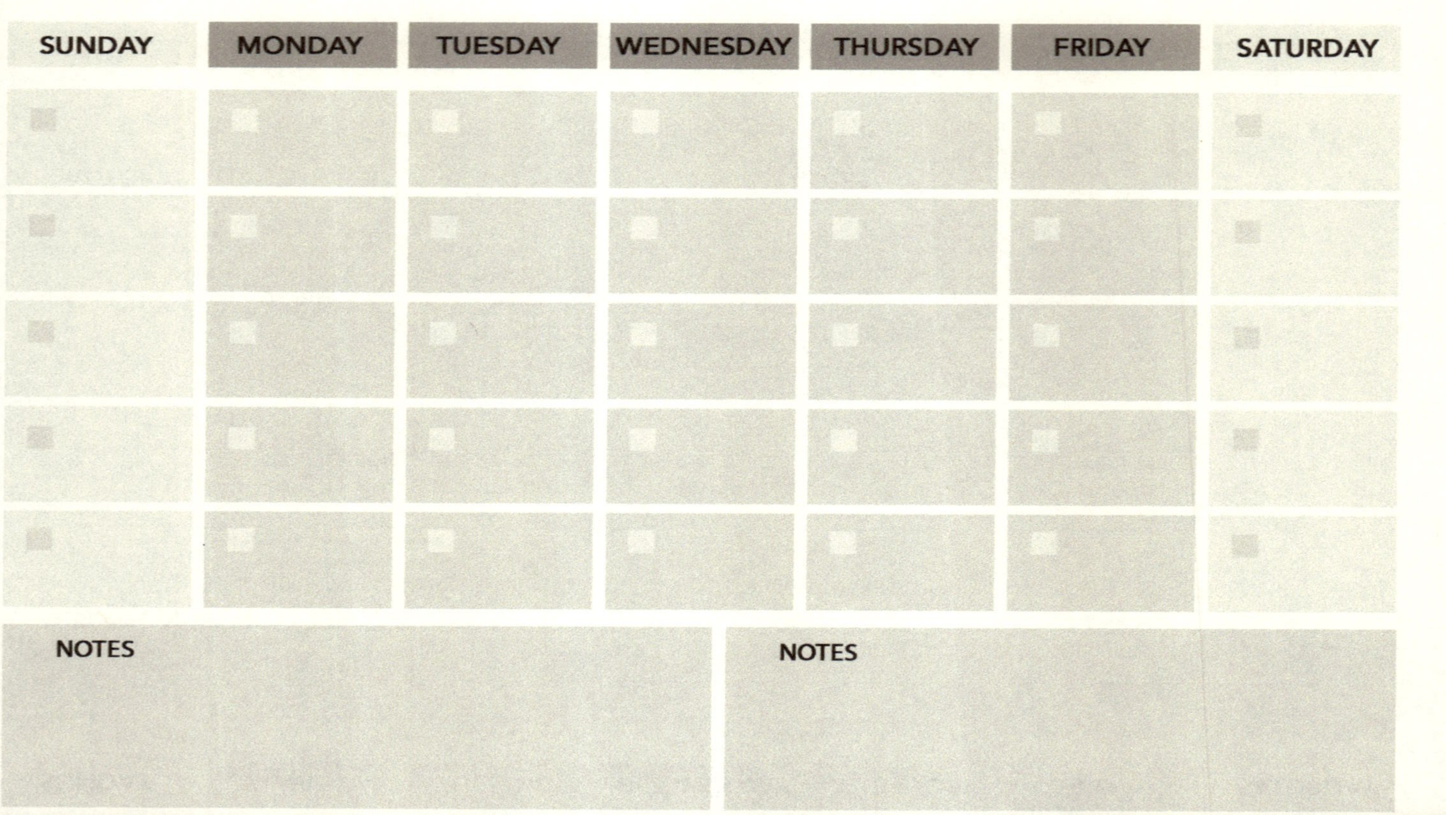

SUNDAY
MONDAY
TUESDAY
WEDNESDAY
THURSDAY
FRIDAY
SATURDAY
NOTES
NOTES

SUNDAY	MONDAY	TUESDAY	WEDNESDAY	THURSDAY	FRIDAY	SATURDAY

NOTES

NOTES

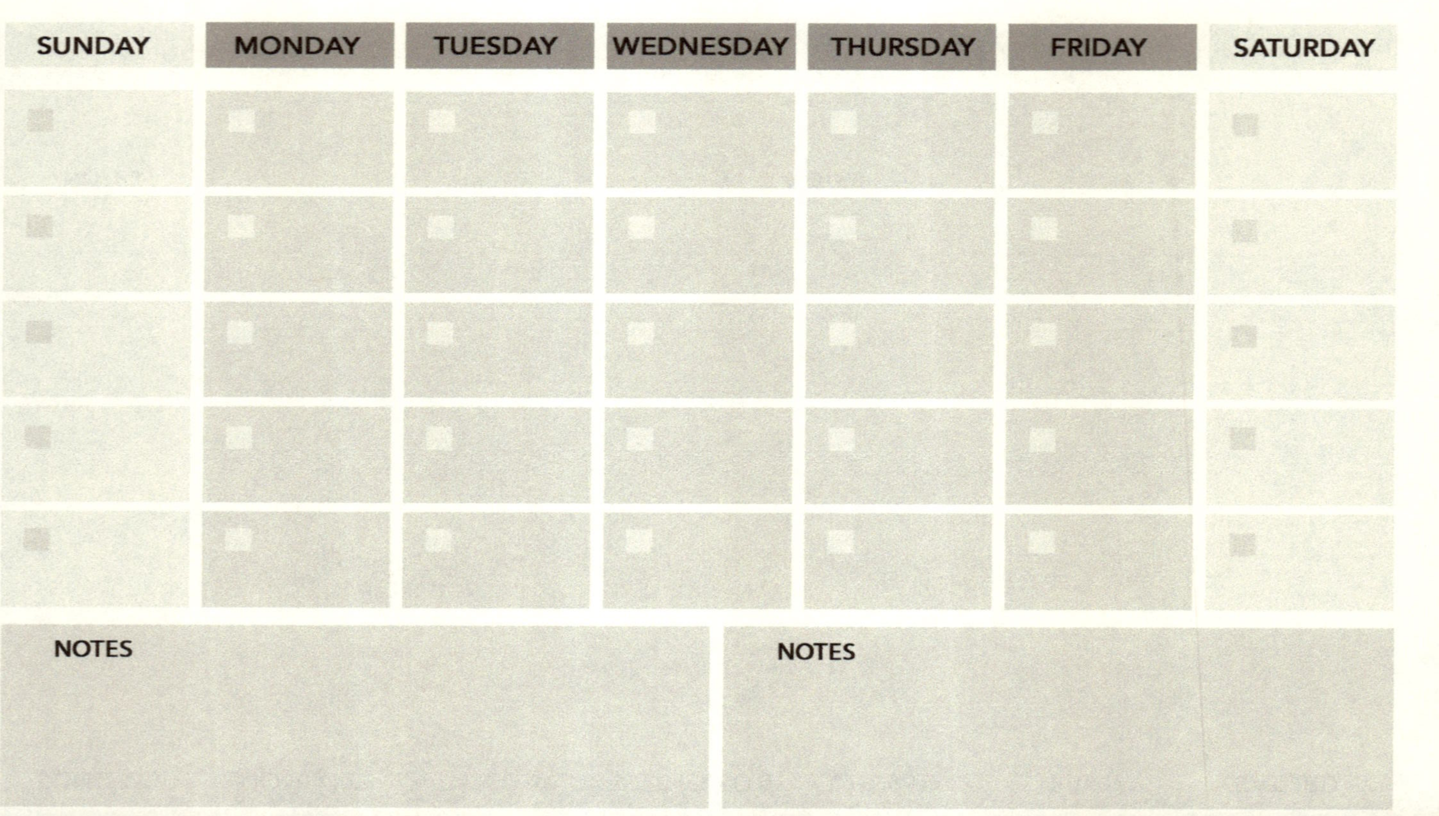

SUNDAY
MONDAY
TUESDAY
WEDNESDAY
THURSDAY
FRIDAY
SATURDAY
NOTES
NOTES

SUNDAY	MONDAY	TUESDAY	WEDNESDAY	THURSDAY	FRIDAY	SATURDAY

NOTES

NOTES

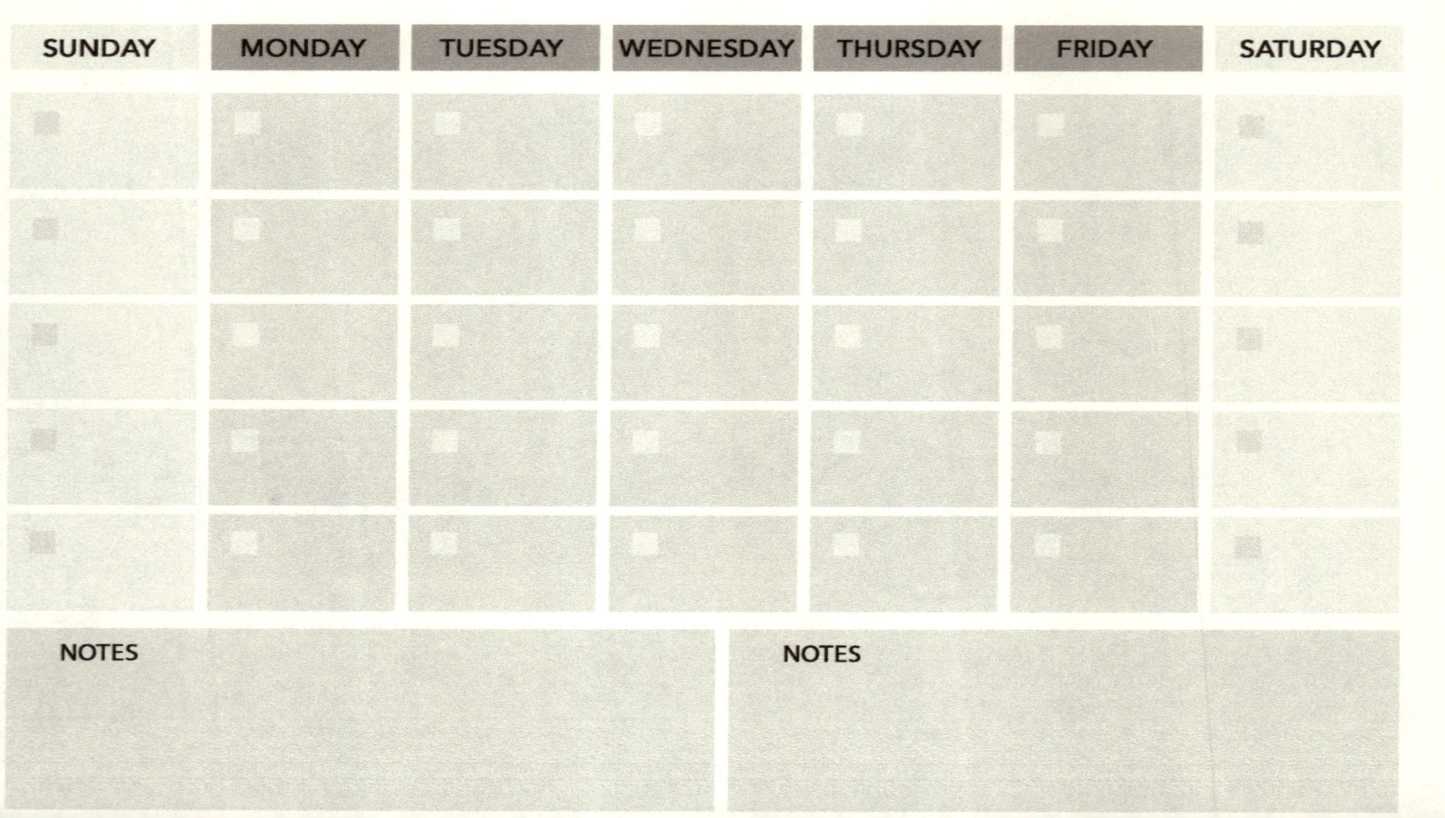

SUNDAY
MONDAY
TUESDAY
WEDNESDAY
THURSDAY
FRIDAY
SATURDAY
NOTES
NOTES

SUNDAY	MONDAY	TUESDAY	WEDNESDAY	THURSDAY	FRIDAY	SATURDAY

NOTES

NOTES

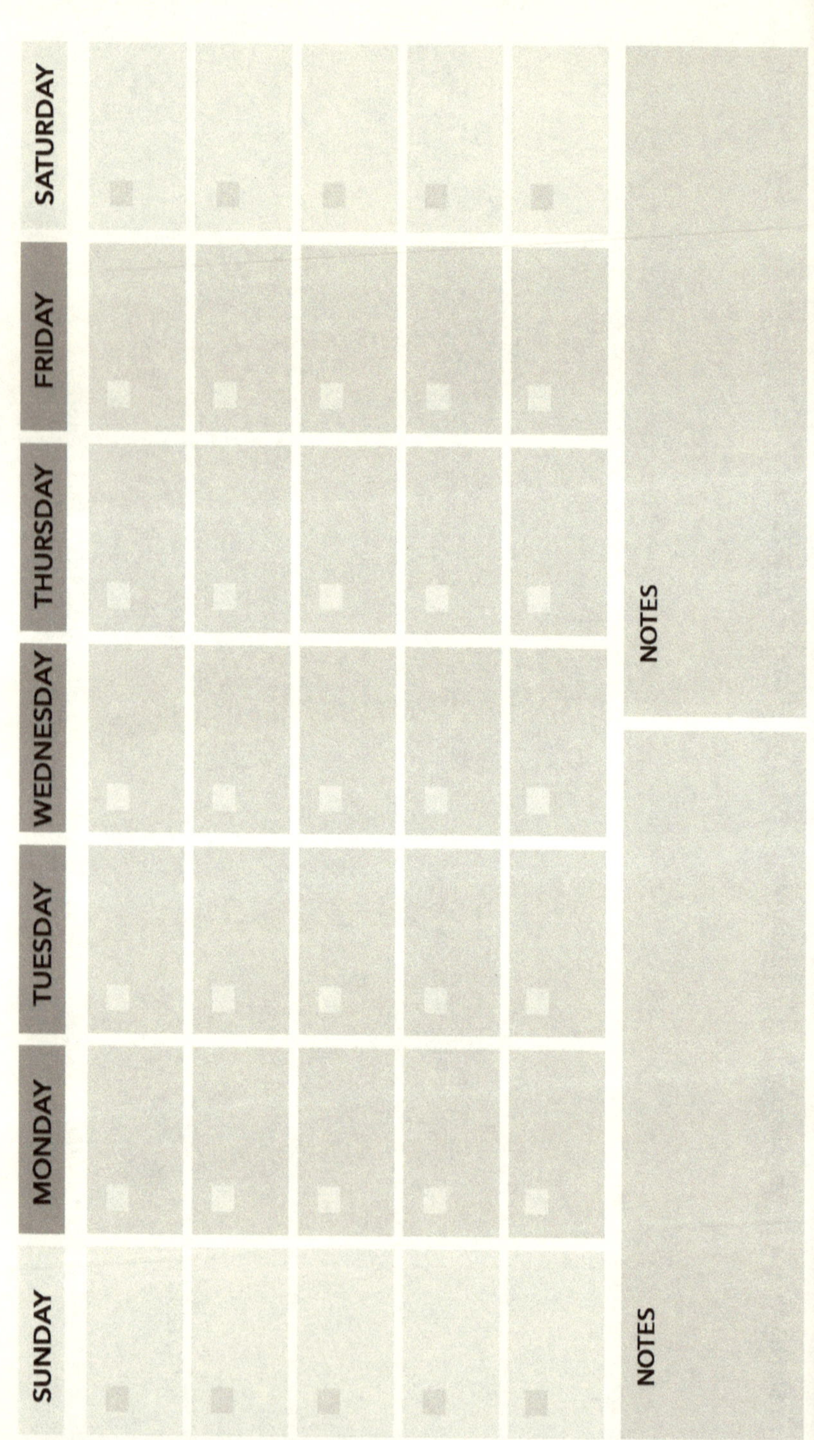

SUNDAY	MONDAY	TUESDAY	WEDNESDAY	THURSDAY	FRIDAY	SATURDAY

NOTES

NOTES

SUNDAY	MONDAY	TUESDAY	WEDNESDAY	THURSDAY	FRIDAY	SATURDAY

NOTES

NOTES

9 798611 259917